Contents

<u>Introduction</u>

This book contains the first two volumes in a series entitled *"The Enlightenment App."* In this book I will describe how I woke up from the relatively unconscious state of mind that I was in for over twenty years and began a much more dynamic phase of my life in which I experience a daily connection with a Universal Consciousness. I will also tell you exactly how I transformed from being someone who was caught up in our cultural matrix, experiencing periodic bouts of fear, depression, uncertainty, and confusion, to someone who has purpose and direction and lives in faith and joy. I don't claim to have all the answers. I am merely a seeker on the path as you most likely are. I did, however, become aware of some truly amazing things that I want to share with you! I am actually able to receive information from a brilliant, evolved consciousness that is beyond the Earth. I believe virtually everyone has the ability to discover their divinely guided purpose and transform their lives and reality into something they love.

In this book I will be discussing the importance of your pineal (pronounced "pie-NEEL" or "PIE-ne-al") gland and how to fix your pineal gland (you didn't know it was broken?!). Healing your pineal gland is such an important issue I'm quite certain I would not be able to receive nearly as much of the information the Universe is currently offering me if I had not restored the health of this gland. I have become friends with many people who travel on the higher paths of enlightenment and the vast majority of them have done similar things to heal their bodies as well. In addition to offering you the information I have regarding your pineal gland, I will provide you with strategies for increasing the amount of melatonin your pineal gland produces. When I first started working as a nutritionist, I thought melatonin was pretty much just something that helped one sleep better. I had heard about the "Pineal Theory of Aging," and I knew there were studies that strongly suggest melatonin levels determine how long mammals live, but I didn't realize just how powerful and amazing melatonin was until I researched the topic. I am very excited to share what I have learned about this melatonin molecule with you! Then, in the last chapter of this book, I will share some information on dimethyltryptamine (DMT) and cannabis that will perhaps help dispel some common misconceptions and misinformation about these substances and provide you with some new ideas to explore.

The concept that there is something beyond our normal, everyday physical experiences here on Earth has been expressed in some of the earliest examples of recorded human history. All the ancient civilizations of Egypt, India, China, and Central and South America left relics depicting various elements of other levels of consciousness. In our world today, many people have stated they can talk with God, see angels, channel entities, or speak with dead people. Others claim to have had Out Of Body experiences, Near Death Experiences (NDE) or say they have clairvoyant, psychic, Remote Viewing or Extra Sensory Perception (ESP) abilities. Many more people who experience these things do not talk about these subjects publicly for fear of ridicule, or worse.

I didn't used to believe in hardly any of this stuff. I was raised catholic, so as a child, I believed in angels and a God, but that's about it. Even then, I figured that I wouldn't be communicating directly with anything like them until after I was dead. Now I know differently. All over the world, people are waking up from relative unconsciousness. Many Quantum Physicists state that this physical dimension is just one part of what actually exists. In fact, most Quantum Physicists believe that approximately

99.9999% of what exists is immaterial; this is based on the idea that objects are composed of atoms and not only is there space between the atoms in objects, but atoms themselves are believed to be more than 99% immaterial. Can you even conceive the thought that virtually nothing in this universe is solid? For now, perhaps it is enough for us to just realize that our brains try to make sense of what our eyes "see" in the limited light spectrum that they can perceive (roughly between 380 nanometer – 740 nanometer) and feed us information that is based on preconceived notions and extrapolation. The desk may feel solid to our hand, but our hand itself is over 99% immaterial.

Perhaps you have already sensed that there is much more to our reality than meets the eye. Perhaps you simply want to explore the possibilities of there being something more than the mainstream societal beliefs of reality. In either case, I invite you to listen to my story with an open mind. My main desire is NOT to convince you of anything through my words but rather to encourage you to put some focused action towards having an awakening of your own or increase your current connection to the Universal Consciousness. In that way, you can have your own knowing and explore the various levels of consciousness as you wish. In this book series, I will describe, in detail, ways in which you can significantly increase your chances of making a stronger connection to the great wireless Universal internet that surrounds us. Enjoy.

Chapter 1: A Lesson in Karma

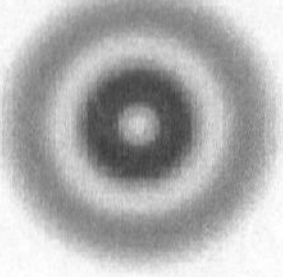

Note to reader: I had to edit out some geographical details in order not to be confessing to a crime here.

It all began one cold night in 1985. I was 18 years old and I lived in [a fairly large city located in New England]. It was Saturday night, and I owned a '77 Thunderbird, so naturally I was cruising on the main street of the city, the "miracle mile." At that time, the downtown portion of this roadway consisted of four lanes, two lanes heading south and two lanes heading north. Sadly, how well my social life was going at that time was strongly contingent on the people who happened to pull up next to me at the red lights. At one particular stoplight, a car containing two males about my age pulled up alongside my car. Since they were not of the exact gender I was interested in, I was about to divert my eyes back to the streetlight in case a car race to the next light was necessary. Before I could completely avert my eyes, however, the young man in the passenger seat of the car produced a small jackknife and proceeded to stare at me while making small stabbing movements with the knife. I was able to shake my head and laugh it off. The light turned green, we proceeded on our way without comparing the horsepower of our cars and eventually we both rolled up to another red light. I was again stopped alongside that same car, and the young man in the passenger seat of the car was again brandishing his knife while staring at me. I gave him more of a hard stare back this time; I wasn't enjoying his joke anymore. He made more exaggerated stabbing motions in the air towards me from inside his friend's car. It was pretty darn cold out, and his window was rolled up, so he couldn't stab too far. I decided that I was going to do something to stop his charade stabs. I put my car in park, opened my car door, got out, took a couple steps toward the car he was in, and banged once on his window with my leather glove wrapped hand to indicate that I was tired of seeing his knife. Unfortunately, my fist didn't just bang on the car's passenger window, but rather went right through it, causing shards of glass to sail into the car towards the knife-wielder's face. I was probably as stunned as he was, but eventually I got back in my car, put it in drive, and got the heck out of there. They chased me for a while, getting very close to my car's bumper, but then raced off in another direction.

Well, that night, and for the weeks that followed, I was fearful. What if they had gotten my license plate number? What if the police had a description of my car and were looking for a metallic green Thunderbird? I decided to avoid cruising the main street for a while. Eventually my fears subsided, and I even started cruising that main street again. I had gotten away with it, a lucky break.

Years went by, and I was determined to make Spring Break 1989 one to remember by flying down to Florida. My brother lived there at the time and I wanted to see what Daytona Beach was like. A coworker of mine at the hotel I was working at part-time wanted to go to Florida as well, so I had a friend to go with and the vacation was on.

The first night in Florida, we decided to head to a dance club in Cocoa Beach. I felt rather stiff and nerdy in this fast-paced, modern club, standing around watching a dance floor competition through my black-framed glasses. Nonetheless, one delightful young woman thought I was cute, or took pity on me, and was actually talking to me. She would walk over, chat with me a bit, and then she'd step back to her friends and look attractive. She spoke with me again and started moving back over towards her friends but was stopped short by a solid young man who leaned in and whispered something in her ear while glaring at me. Well, it wasn't long before I was asking the girl what he had said, and she told me that he had told her that I had a sexually transmitted disease. I decided that I wasn't going to tolerate him telling her that. I marched my 140-pound body right over to 6 foot him and told him to shut the hell up. He just drew his face into a snarl and acted aloof. A couple of minutes went by, and some more dancers were putting on a show, but I couldn't help noticing something out of the very corner of my eye; it was 6 foot's fist coming right at my head. He would've punched me right on the side of the head, but since I turned my head to look, his fist struck my glasses, popping the right lens out and jamming it against my face. The lens cut my right eyebrow, and it started to bleed. The young man then pretended that he had done nothing and turned to watch the dance show. I stood there stunned for several seconds as a few drops of blood dripped down from my eyebrow. As I stood watching him, it occurred to me that he was no longer watching me. My ego told me that I could beat him up, and I charged at him and hurled a fist at his face, striking him on the cheekbone. He reeled off to one side and then started running towards the front exit. Blinded with rage, I pursued him as quickly as I could.

To make a long story shorter, there was a police officer at the front of the club and I shouted for the officer to grab this guy. My testimony, along with the testimony of several other people in the bar who had seen him throw his punch, got this person in jail for the night. My friend drove me in our rented Mustang to the closest hospital to get the gash in my right eyebrow stitched up. The hospital staff stitched me up and before long, we were back in the Mustang.

As my friend was driving me back to my brother's house, I asked my companion if he had ever had to get stitches. He told me that one night he was cruising [the main street of our hometown] and a guy put his fist through the window of the car he was in, causing pieces of glass to fly towards his face. The glass had lacerated the right side of his face and he had to go to the hospital and get some stitches. Well, you could've knocked me over with a feather. After a pause, I said "Was he a big guy?" and he responded, "Well, he had a Marines bumper sticker on the back of his car." I had a Marines bumper sticker on the back of my Thunderbird because I had bought the car from a man who had left town to become a Marine. This person driving the car I was in was the young man with the jackknife. There I was, riding in a car on a lonely stretch of road in Florida, about 2000 miles and four years away from my car-punching incident, and the person driving the car was the same person who had that jackknife that night. Not only that, but he had just taken me to a hospital to get stitches in my face caused by glass hitting my face due to a punch that should've never been thrown. He was the same young man that had to go to the hospital to get stitches because I threw a punch that should've never been thrown, which caused glass to cut his face. I didn't say much the rest of the way back to my brother's house. I had always thought that this buddy of mine seemed somehow familiar to me the first time I met him, but I had never been able to figure out why until that minute. I never told him that I was the person who punched that car window in, and as far as I know, he never knew I was that person. The next day we drove to the University of Florida in Gainesville because he wanted to meet up with a friend he had gone to high school with. I'm nearly certain this friend of his was the person driving the car that I punched that night in 1985. This young man wanted to drive our rented Mustang, so he drove, my buddy was in the passenger seat, and I was now a silent passenger in the back seat of *their* car.

This incident convinced me that there might be some kind of invisible law or force affecting my life. Some people would say that these events were merely a coincidence, but I've since learned that "coincidences" are important! Back in 1989, I didn't even know what the word "karma" meant, but that's when I first started truly believing that some force in the Universe existed that gives me back whatever I put out. There are other expressions for this force: "cause and effect," "what you sow, so shall you reap," "give what you want to receive." This was an amazing concept for my young mind to wrap itself around. I had been conditioned by my schooling and society to place great importance on rational thought and left-brained thinking. I had majored in computer science in college and what's more linear thinking than that? Nonetheless, I felt as though I had no choice but to accept the distinct possibility that there was this invisible force or law that can influence my life. I also had to allow for the possibility that there may even be more than one of these invisible laws or forces [There are 3 main laws in this physical dimension: 1) You are Existence, 2) What you put out you get back, 3) The One is All and the All is One].

Well, years went by, and I got distracted and consumed by everyday life. Although I was still afraid of doing anything wrong that might cause me "bad karma," I wasn't any more enlightened or intuitive than the average person [Karma should NOT be viewed as a "punishment" or "reparation." Its purpose is to direct people back toward their paths of learning and useful experience]. I was more honest and ethical than most of my peers, but I didn't have any special insight on things. In fact, I had shifted from believing the tenets of the Catholic Church that I had been raised with to becoming an atheist; my college philosophy professors had made me question the logic of believing in a God. I looked around me at the world, saw many problems with it, and concluded that God either failed or didn't even exist; in either case, God deserved no worship from me.

In 1993, I moved from New England to California. I like sunny, warm weather and New England wasn't supplying enough of that. I didn't know anyone in California, didn't have a job lined up, and I didn't know where I was going to stay, but I flew into Lindbergh Field, San Diego's International Airport, with some luggage and about $3,000 of hard-earned money in the bank. It took me a lot of time and energy to find a place to live, get a job and build a life for myself out in California. I was in my late twenty's now, and my main concerns were money, women, and partying. During my thirties, I found myself working at the same place for years and dating the same woman, whom I had grown apart from and fallen out of love with. I spent most of my free time playing or studying chess; I would often spend over three hours playing a single game of chess against a chess computer. I was in a miserable rut. I needed a miracle to wake me up.

Chapter 2: The Accident?

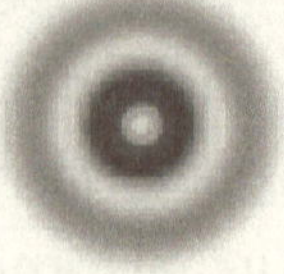

On June 27th, 1998, I was driving my Saturn sedan on Mission Valley Freeway 8 East in San Diego. I was taking a two-lane exit towards Fairmount Avenue when another driver attempted to pass through my lane to enter the ramp leading to Escondido Freeway 15 North. The driver struck the front panel of my Saturn causing my car to go into a spin and my airbag to deploy. The airbag knocked both of my hands off the steering wheel and completely obstructed my view. My car spun around and I crashed into a concrete divider while going backwards at about 50 miles per hour. My car flipped into the air and the last thing I remember seeing is the asphalt rushing towards my windshield as my car was plummeting roof-first towards the ground. I woke up to the sound of someone screaming at me. I was hanging upside down by my seatbelt. My head and neck were bent against the roof, which was now like the floor. My knee was bleeding, my elbow was bleeding, and I had glass stuck in various parts of my body. I looked over at my passenger, the woman that I was dating, and she was unconscious. I yelled at her until she thankfully opened her eyes and regained consciousness. We crawled out of the holes where our side windows used to be to find that a large group of people had gathered; some were civilians, some were police, and some were paramedics. I was really confused as to how they had all just appeared there. I didn't realize that I had been unconscious for many minutes (I don't know how long I was unconscious). I tried to stand up, but I fell back down. The paramedics placed me and my girlfriend on stretchers. She fared better than I did, but $4,925.31 later I was released from Mercy Hospital.

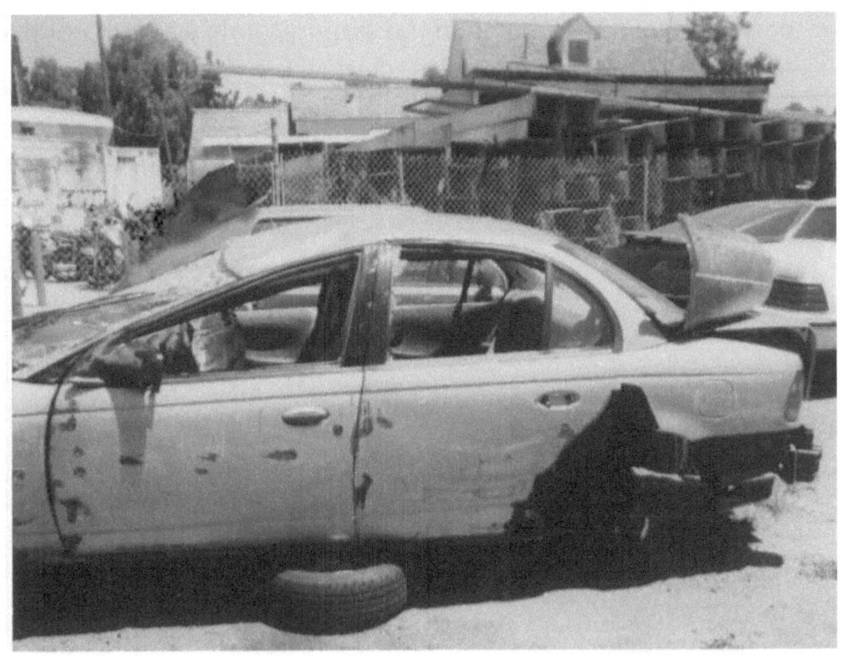

My Saturn at a junkyard after the accident.

My life was quite unpleasant after that accident. My spine had been compressed and the muscles in my back were on their way to healing wrong. I was given Naproxen to reduce my muscle swelling. I could barely stand up and couldn't go in to work. The pain and discomfort were very real. I sunk into depression. I developed panic attacks, irritable bowel syndrome, and agoraphobia (the fear of large, public places). I became too afraid to drive on freeways. I started being afraid to even be home alone, but I was alone more than ever because my girlfriend left me. I was feeling so depressed that I decided to spend nearly all the money I had left to undergo laser eye surgery. I had always wanted to have perfect vision, but I was always too afraid to undergo the procedure. Now I had the perfect plan; if they botched the surgery, and I was blind or even partially blind, I could just kill myself.

Chapter 3: My First Conversation with a Higher Being

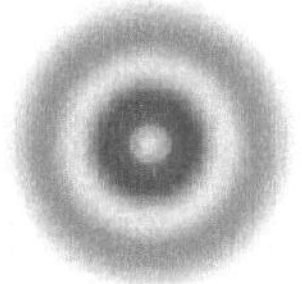

I had the laser eye surgery performed and my eyes were healing
fine. I had been spending a lot of time in my apartment because
my back hurt, and I didn't have the urge to do much of anything.
I was alone with my thoughts most of the time. I would lie in
bed, even during daylight hours, and just let my mind wander. I
was becoming increasingly concerned that the mountain lions at
Cuyamaca Rancho State Park were going to be hunted down and
killed because they had occasionally attacked or threatened
people who were on the land the mountain lions lived on. I was
giving serious thought to the idea of devoting my life to
protecting mountain lions. I decided to take a shower, and then
it happened. As I was taking a shower I was asking, aloud,
"What should I DO with my life?!"…and to my GREAT surprise I
got an answer. A voice said to me [please note that I am
paraphrasing all of this to the best of my recollection] "don't
waste your life trying to fix one aspect of creation, a true creator
can do in an instant things that [the current] you couldn't get
done in a lifetime." I "heard" the words mostly inside of my
head, but the shower radio was actually broadcasting some of
the entity's words as well. I thought that maybe I was just
imagining things, but my mind quickly formed another question.
"Well, what SHOULD I do with my life then?!" Again, I heard the
voice, it replied, "You should LIVE your life and enjoy it."
"Really?" I countered in disbelief, "That's all I need to do?"

"Yes," the voice replied, "I want you to be happy. I'm happy when you're happy."

I was glad to hear such upbeat messages, and a wave of gratefulness washed over me but at the same time, I was shaken to the point of trembling. I was overcome with humility and a sense of inferiority in the presence of this higher being. In fact, despite the fact that I seemed to be able to have any question I asked answered, even questions that I had had since I was a young boy, I essentially invited this God-like being to leave. I just felt so unworthy of His [yes, I did feel a decidedly "male" energy] attention. I felt as though a great spotlight was shining down upon me from above this Earth, which exposed me and made me visible to the entire Universe. I said "Okay, thank you, thank you... that's all I need, thank you" while mentally wishing that IT would just leave me be. I could feel IT graciously complying, but then a song started playing on my shower radio that had the lyric "God is dead" in it. I burst out laughing because I suddenly realized there was absolutely no mistake that that song was playing. In a heartbeat, I was made to understand that not only did this higher being have a sense of humor, but I also realized that humor is actually a divine gift intended to delight us. HE found a way to relieve my fears and insecurities instantly by imparting my body with the vibration of laughter and joy.

Well, there are many things I could say about that conversation, but what I want to make clear to you is that part of the reason I know that I wasn't just "talking with myself" is because the answers I received weren't the type of things that I would've come up with on my own, especially at that time in my life. Although I had a sense of karma, I didn't really believe in God or higher beings at that time. Even the idea that life is meant to be enjoyed was something that had been beaten out of me a long time ago. When I was young, my father asked me, "What do you want to be when you grow up?" to which I replied, "I want to be happy." I remember him reacting to my answer by cynically imitating me while saying "Happy, happy, happy, all I want is to be happy!" as he outwardly showed his disgust with my silly, childish answer [I have since spoken with my dad about this, about 30 years after he said this to me and told him, in a very delicate way, how his words had negatively affected me. I was then able to fully "forgive" him and love him even more, which unblocked a MAJOR energy blockage to joy in my body]. Many of my life experiences, from my middle school years all the way until that day I got into that shower stall with terrible back pain, seemed to confirm to me that life wasn't meant to be enjoyed [I'm certain that this entity would not have told me to pursue what makes me happy if I were someone who took pleasure in doing harmful things]. In addition, I had decided a few years earlier that a "God" would probably be beyond gender. The idea that a God would just be of one gender didn't make sense to me because it seemed to imply that IT would need a God of another gender to complete itself. For several years before this shower event, whenever I spoke with someone about God, I would refer to "Him" as "It." Now, I realize that it wasn't "God" that I spoke with that day anyway, but I didn't know that at the time.

After this contact experience, my life transformed. I began developing a deeper connection to the Universe. I cured myself of Irritable Bowel Syndrome, panic attacks, agoraphobia, major depression, and driving fears, and then began helping thousands of other people overcome these problems by working as a nutritional advisor and writing books about how to cure these conditions. After hurting for about 4 years my back suddenly got fixed one day when I rotated my torso while getting a 5-gallon jug of water out of my car. I felt some muscles in my back tear and this time my back healed correctly. I can now do deadlifts and I still have 20-20 vision. I met and married a loving woman, and at one point I had two kids, three dogs, three cats, four chickens, a rabbit, a bearded dragon, several fish, and a yard full of trees and plants to love. I started receiving information and direction from the Universe nearly every night and when I truly need to, I am allowed to call out to and speak directly with a caring, benevolent being that watches over this part of the Universe. However, the biggest difference in my life has been the sheer amount of joy, love, peace, ease, and happiness that my connection to Source has brought into my body and mind. Before, I was moody, jealous, angry, fearful, whiny, often depressed, and occasionally low-energy, and now, for the most part (not always), I am in a joyful, cheerful, loving, giving, forgiving place of peaceful faith. I feel as though my entire life is being guided, and I feel as though I have found my life's purpose by intuitively serving others.

I need to emphasis that I didn't go straight from "talking to a higher being in the shower" to a wonderful life. I went through a slow metamorphosis, which took over 13 years. One of the main reasons that I'm writing this book is to help speed the progress of anyone who has recently begun traveling on his or her personal road to enlightenment, or to get someone who is just considering transforming their life to get off the proverbial fence and start running down a nearby pathway. As far as I can understand, the main reason that I was able to have that conversation in the shower in 1998 was because a Being decided to contact me because it took pity on me and/or desired [or was required] to help me because my path was so off course. It decided to contact ME. I wasn't able to contact IT. That has changed. Back in 1998, my body, mind, and belief system would never have allowed me to initiate the actualization of such a conversation. One thing that I did have going for me in 1998 is that many of the ways in which I defined myself in this world had been stripped away from me, leaving me mostly undefined.

Many of the societal labels that I defined myself by didn't apply to me anymore: boyfriend, weightlifter, employee, confident, freeway driver, healthy, active. This caused my ego to collapse, allowing me to be more receptive to receiving advice from anyone or anything. I don't think that many people reading this would want to make their life horrible to get some divine advice, and fortunately, that is NOT what's required to acquire a guided life. Through a series of specific actions and practices, I have become able to receive guidance on a daily basis. I have had more direct discussions with this Being that watches over me, and I will tell you about some of the other amazing things this "watchoverer" has told me. But remember, my purpose is not for you to take my word for it or live vicariously through me. My desire is for YOU to experience your own "unbelievable" events for yourself. So with that in mind, please allow me to tell you about *your* built-in Enlightenment App, your pineal gland.

Chapter 4: The Importance of your Pineal Gland to Consciousness

In order for a radio receiver to pull in a specific radio station the radio must be in good working order, have the power to operate, be set to the correct frequency, and have an antenna that is able to receive that particular radio signal (or be located very close to that radio station). In order for YOU to receive information from the Universal Consciousness you need to have a functional receptor, enough power [and space for new energy] in your body, and the correct focus and allowance in your mind. Your pineal gland is like your receptor, your built-in Enlightenment App.

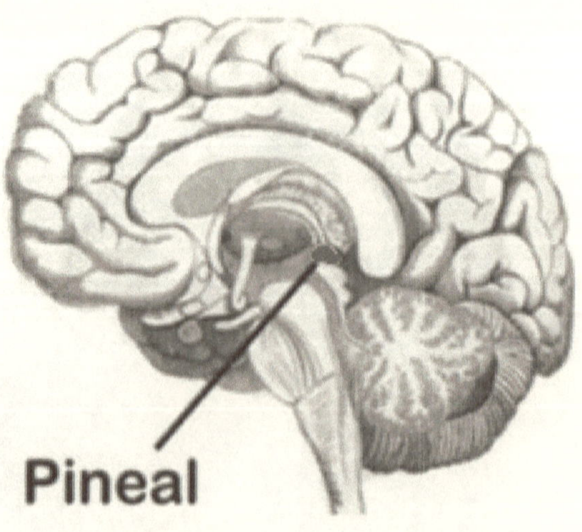

The pineal gland is the first gland to be formed in a human being and is visible in the fetus just three weeks after conception. This gland is shaped like a pine cone and is an outgrowth of the roof of the forebrain located in the exact center of your brain between the two hemispheres. Many scientists believe vertebrate pineal cells share a common evolutionary ancestor with retinal [eye] cells. The structure of the pineal gland is similar to the structure of the cornea, lens, and retina. Many people consider the pineal gland to represent the "third eye" [ajna] chakra. Others believe your "crown" chakra can extend down to your pineal gland and allow pure energy to flow into your body. The third eye chakra is usually depicted as being located in the center of your forehead, and your crown chakra is at the top of your head. These chakras are associated with intuition, imagination, visualization, bliss, self-mastery, and extra sensory perception (ESP). I use a series of colors and tones, along with regularly performing chi gung (also known as Qigong), to strengthen my chakras, but I'll talk more about that in future volumes in this series.

In some vertebrates, such as human beings, the pineal gland is associated with the circadian rhythms of your body [a daily rhythmic activity cycle based on 24-hour intervals]. Even though your pineal gland is located in the center of your brain, this "third eye" synchronizes to the light your body is exposed to. The stimulus derived from light striking the retinas in your eyes travels down your optic nerves to the suprachiasmatic nucleus (SCN) in your hypothalamus that communicates its interpretation of circadian rhythms to your pineal gland. Your pineal gland then uses this information to dictate when it will release the amazing substance known as melatonin into every cell of your body. Although your pineal gland is located in your brain it is NOT protected by the blood-brain barrier and experiences considerable blood flow, second only to your kidneys.

Why should you care about your pineal gland?

Throughout the last few thousand years, the pineal gland has been considered to be a "receptor" by many philosophers and spiritual practitioners; many people consider your pineal gland to be a signal receiver. The ancient Greeks believed their pineal glands connected them to the "Realms of Thought," and the Egyptians used the Eye of Horus to symbolize the third eye in one's head.

Rene Descartes, the famous French scientist and philosopher, believed the pineal gland was the chief interpreter of vision and the "seat of the human soul." In 1644, Descartes created this woodcut to emphasis the importance of the pineal gland:

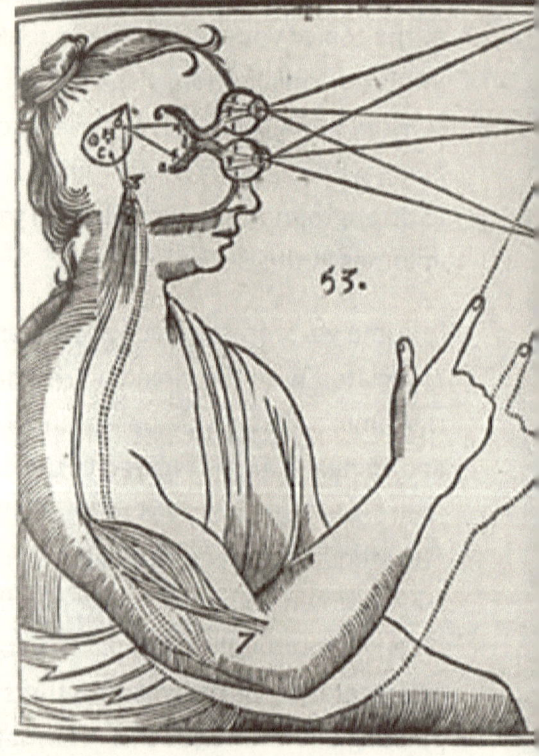

A quote attributed to Descartes reads, "...soul and body touch each other only at a single point, the pineal gland in the head."

Many religions and groups have objects or pictures that depict a pine cone, a common symbolic image of the pineal gland. There is a courtyard in Vatican City called Cortile della Pigna (Courtyard of the Pine Cone), that features a large bronze sculpture of a pine cone which many scholars believe is meant to represent the pineal gland.

Well, no matter what people through the ages believed about this gland I have something that I am living to share with you: I was not able to form a solid connection with the Universal Consciousness until I healed my pineal gland. Everything really started for me, on a daily basis, after I healed this gland.

Chapter 5: The Importance of your Pineal Gland to Your Health

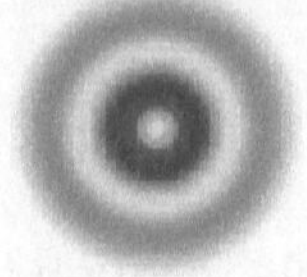

The health of your pineal gland has a strong correlation with how many years you live.

In 1994, Vladimir Lesnikov (et al.), at the Russian Academy of Medical Science in St. Petersburg, performed a study that concluded that when the pineal glands of old mice were transplanted into younger mice, the younger mice experienced a shortened life span (they lived about 17 months). When the pineal glands of young mice were transplanted into older mice, the older mice experienced an increased lifespan (about 34 months on average). Studies have also demonstrated the life-extension possibilities of melatonin specifically and the pineal gland is responsible for most of the production of melatonin in your body.

According to Dr. Lesnikov, "Circadian [nighttime], chronic administration of melatonin and young-to-old pineal grafting into the thymus have provided evidence for the existence of an endogenous, primary and central "aging clock" in the pineal gland. The new model described here serves to definitely demonstrate that the replacement of the pineal gland of an old mouse with the pineal from a young, syngeneic donor mouse remarkably prolongs its life and, conversely, the "old" pineal transplanted into a younger mouse will considerably shorten its life span. Pineal cross-transplantation thus provides clear-cut evidence for the central role of the pineal gland in the initiation and progression of senescence [biological aging]. It offers a novel basis for interventions in the aging process."

The results of these studies were further interpreted by Dr. Russel J. Reiter, at the University of Texas Health Science Center's Department of Cellular and Structural Biology located in San Antonio, Texas. Dr. Reiter stated, "Within recent years, many investigators have implicated the pineal gland and melatonin in the processes of both aging and age-related diseases. These theories stem from the importance of melatonin in a number of biological functions and the fact that melatonin production in the organism is gradually lost throughout life, such that in very old individuals of any species the circadian melatonin rhythm is barely discernible. In most species, from algae to humans, where it has been investigated, melatonin has been shown to exhibit a strong circadian rhythm in production and secretion, with high levels of the indole always being associated with the dark period of the light/dark cycle. One theory states when the melatonin rhythm deteriorates during aging, other circadian rhythms are likewise weakened and rhythms become desynchronized. This desynchronization is believed to contribute significantly to aging and to render animals more susceptible to age-related diseases. Another theory assumes the waning melatonin cycle provides an important switch for genetically programmed aging at the cellular level; furthermore, because all cells in the organism are exposed to the same gradually dampening melatonin signal throughout life, all cells age more or less at the same rate. In this theory, it is presumed to be the duration of the nocturnally elevated melatonin (which, like the amplitude, is reduced during aging), which, when coupled to a time-gating signal, is consequential in determining the rate of aging. Another compelling argument that the reduction in melatonin with age may be contributory to aging and the onset of age-related diseases is based on the recent observation that melatonin is the most potent hydroxyl radical scavenger thus far discovered. A prominent theory of aging attributes the rate of aging to accumulated free radical damage. Inasmuch as melatonin can markedly protect macromolecules, especially DNA, against free radical attack, it could, indeed, be a major factor in determining the rate at which organisms age. Besides its ability to scavenge the highly toxic hydroxyl radical, melatonin also promotes the activity of the antioxidative enzyme glutathione peroxidase, thereby further reducing oxidative damage. These actions may be manifested more obviously in the central nervous system, which is highly susceptible to damage by oxygen-based radicals and, because of its inability to regenerate and its high vulnerability to oxidative attack, its deterioration may be especially important in aging." [Reiter, R. The aging pineal gland and its physiological consequences. Bioessays. 14(3):169-175, 1992]

According to Walter Pierpaoli and Vladimir Lesnikov, the pineal gland controls your neuroendocrine function and helps your immune system "recognize and react against any noxious, endogenous, or exogenous agent." When pineal function is turned off, the result is senescence [biological aging]. Many of the diseases of aging reflect this progressive decline of the self-recognition capacity that can be seen through the "emergence of peripheral desynchronization [loss of integrated functioning of the neuroendocrine system and shifting of youthful homeostatic conditions] and [promotion of] autoimmune, anaplastic, neoplastic, and degenerative processes." Melatonin may address the core of these problems.

Because of these studies an entire Pineal Theory of Aging has developed. Your pineal gland regulates your entire body's hormone balance. During the day, your pineal gland produces melatonin (but only secretes significant amounts of it at night) and produces and secretes 5-methoxytryptophol and other hormones and chemicals that haven't even been named yet. 5-methoxytryptophol helps to preserve membrane fluidity in the liver during times of oxidative stress. Studies also suggest that melatonin helps the mitochondria in your cells produce ATP (cell energy) and maintain a desirable homeostasis [Pandi-Perumal, S. Melatonin Antioxidative Defense: Therapeutical Implications for Aging and Neurodegenerative Processes. Neurotoxicity Research 23(3):267-300 June 2013]. Other studies suggest your pineal gland helps to maintain your immune system and regulate the function of your thymus gland. After reviewing much of the research data we have concerning the pineal gland and its effect on the long-term health of one's body, I am convinced one's health and natural lifespan is directly related to how healthy one's pineal gland is.

Chapter 6: Why your Pineal Gland is probably Damaged

If you live in the United States, or anywhere else where the water is fluoridated, there is very high chance your pineal gland has been damaged.

In 1997, a study conducted at the University of Surrey in England proposed that fluoride accumulates in, and damages, the pineal gland. The study also suggested that fluoride interferes with the pineal gland's production of melatonin.

Water fluoridation was introduced to the United States in the 1940s as a way to dispose of the hazardous waste products left over from the manufacture of aluminum. This waste product, known as sodium fluoride, cost the aluminum manufacturers a lot of money to dispose of properly and they were coming under increasing pressure from nearby ranchers to handle their fluoride problem as it was causing harm to cattle and farmland. They found their problem conveniently solved when they were allowed to sell their waste to cities that put the fluoride into the municipal water supply. About 70% of the "tap" water in the United States is fluoridated and fluoride is also added to most toothpastes, many mouth rinses, and is found in foods that are sprayed with fluoride-based pesticides or washed in fluoride-contaminated water.

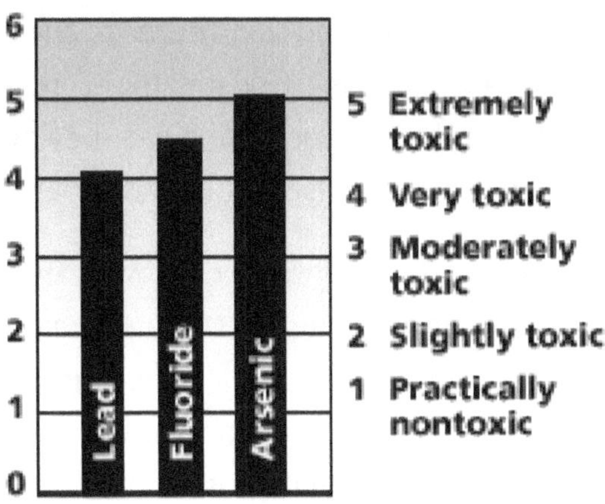

Nowadays, most of the fluoride in tap water is sodium silicofluoride, a waste product of the phosphate fertilizer industry. In addition to its own inherent toxicity, this waste product may also contain other byproducts such as arsenic, lead, cadmium, and mercury. Studies have shown fluoride can actually increase the accumulation of lead in your body, even facilitating the transport of heavy metals into your brain. A review of the effects fluoride has on human intelligence found 18 studies that strongly suggested intelligence decreases in correlation with higher fluoride exposure (Connett, M. and Limeback, H., 2008).

You might think, "If fluoride is so bad for me I would learn about this from the news." Well there are many reasons why you don't hear much about the fact hydrofluosilicic acid, fluosilicic acid, and sodium fluoride are all categorized as hazardous waste. First, almost all mainstream media [television news and programs, online news and entertainment pages, magazines, movies, newspapers, and radio news and programs] is owned and controlled by just six companies [Comcast, Time Warner, The Walt Disney Company, Rupert Murdock's News Corporation, AT&T, and CBS]. These companies are not required to report information that does not serve their interests, and some people believe these companies routinely distort the truth to protect the revenues of the various other companies they own (such as the multi-billion-dollar phosphate fertilizer companies).

One might also believe their dentist would warn them about fluoride instead of recommending it. Dentists are only taught about the "benefits" of fluoride in college, just as they are taught about the "benefits" of x-rays and amalgam fillings (even though there is no question radiation is a contributing factor to cancer and amalgam fillings contain toxic mercury). There is strong evidence that, in the past, research showing the various negative effects of fluoride was routinely "whitewashed." There have been documented cases where researchers who performed studies that demonstrated a "negative" effect from fluoride were fired from their jobs. Scientists, dentists, and others who have publically spoken out about the potential toxicity of fluoride have also been punished. Dr. William Marcus, the former chief toxicologist for the United States Environmental Protection Agency Office of Drinking Water, lost his job in 1991 after he insisted that fluoride was a cancer-causing agent [a carcinogen]. Marcus eventually proved his case in court and was reinstated. In 1991, an investigation by the Senate Environment and Public Works Committee showed government scientists had been prevented from showing a finding that portrayed fluoride more as a toxin than a helpful substance. For more proof fluoride is toxic just look on the label of any toothpaste containing fluoride. By law, they must put a warning similar to this on the label:

"WARNING: KEEP OUT OF REACH OF CHILDREN. IF YOU ACCIDENTALLY SWALLOW MORE THAN USED FOR BRUSHING, SEEK PROFESSIONAL ASSISTANCE OR CONTACT A POISON CONTROL CENTER IMMEDIATELY."

Some of the health consequences of too much fluoride include:

Dental fluorosis (which is indicated by loss of teeth enamel and white or tan spots on teeth)

Tooth decay (due to fluoride increasing the body's retention of lead that can lead to tooth decay)

Infertility in both men and women

Gastritis

Increased risk of hypothyroidism

Kidney and liver damage

Bone damage and increased risk of fractures

Brain damage, decreased attention span, and lowering of intelligence

Increased risk of cancer (Ramesh, N., et al., 2001)

Dying at a younger age (Machoy-Mokrzynska, A., 2004)

Getting back to the subject of fluoride possibly affecting your pineal gland (and even enlightenment itself!), doctor Jennifer Luke, of the University of Surrey in England, stated fluoride accumulates in the pineal gland more than in any other soft tissue in the body (Luke, J 1997, 2001). In fact, the level of fluoride can get so high (~300 ppm) that it is capable of inhibiting the production of critical enzymes. Furthermore, the hard tissue of the pineal gland accumulates more fluoride (up to 21,000 ppm) than any other hard tissue (even teeth and bone) in the body. Dr. Luke also found that animals subjected to fluoride had reduced levels of melatonin metabolites, which indicates lower levels of circulating melatonin. According to Dr. Luke,

"...the human pineal gland contains the highest concentration of fluoride in the body. Fluoride is associated with depressed pineal melatonin synthesis."

Many people who are aware of the potential dangers of fluoride are convinced it's being purposely added to the water supply to either "dumb people down," keep them "under control" [the active ingredient in Prozac is fluoxetine hydrochloride, a chemical compound containing fluoride], or control overpopulation. Some people believe fluoride is added to water and products to harm our pineal glands and prevent people from having spiritual awakenings that would allow them to see the cultural matrix more objectively. I will leave those ideas for you to investigate. Just be aware that water fluoridation has actually been outlawed in many countries.

For more information on fluoride, I suggest you read *The Fluoride Deception* by Christopher Bryson. Mr. Bryson discusses some of the ways in which politics, industry, and the military have expedited the addition of fluoride into drinking water.

Even if you haven't been subjected to fluoride, studies show calcium phosphate crystals usually form in the pineal gland over time causing your pineal gland to become "calcified" (that's not a good thing). Most studies on this matter show that by age 18 most people's pineal glands have become calcified. Many people's pineal glands are so calcified that the gland looks like a solid piece of calcium on magnetic resonance imaging (MRI) scans. This fact led one seeker of awareness to write, "Give me back my soft pineal gland so I can dream like I did as a child. Vivid, lucid dreams, all the time. It was like my imagination was much more vivid and creative. I'm starting to believe that it [was] not because I was young and naive; my pineal gland was full of the good stuff."

The primary causes of calcification include calcium supplements, halides [chlorine, bromide, and fluoride], calcium added to processed foods and supplements [such as calcium phosphate, calcium carbonate, and dicalcium phosphate], calcifying substances in tap water, and a diet that causes systemic body acidity. Most people in America are eating the Standard American Diet (SAD), which is high in fat, refined sugars (especially corn syrup), hydrogenated oils, and flours and grains, all of which causes their bodies to become acidic. People are often told to increase their calcium intake in an attempt to reduce their acidity and "keep their bones strong," but without adequate magnesium, boron, silica, and potassium (all of which the majority of people are deficient in) calcium supplements can do more damage than they fix.

I personally believe eating a healthy, nutrient-dense diet and avoiding the toxic ingredients found in the diets of the vast majority of people in developed countries is so important that I have devoted myself to being a nutritionist and have written books on how to heal and empower your entire body by eating the right foods and avoiding the numerous harmful ones. Many people who seek enlightenment regard their bodies as temples that hold their spirit and believe the "cleaner they eat" (the less chemicals/toxins they ingest) the easier it is for them to stay connected with divine guidance. When I switched from the typical American diet of processed foods to a primarily whole foods diet, both my physical and spiritual lives improved tremendously. Good, wholesome food gives your body the energy to power up your "radio" receiver as well as gives you the energy to do whatever you want to do in life! If you're interested in using food to increase the life force in your physical body, please consider reading the next book in this Enlightenment App series entitled, "How to Use Food to Help You Be Healthy, Happy, and Increase Your Chi."

Chapter 7: Healing and Strengthening your Pineal Gland

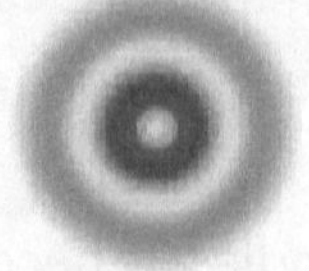

There are many ways you can help heal your pineal gland. The first thing you should do is reduce or eliminate anything that may harm your pineal gland. I would recommend trying to eliminate fluoride from your life. I have installed a fluoride-reducing filter on the water line that feeds into my refrigerator, and I pretty much only drink water that has been filtered through a reverse-osmosis filter (I add beneficial minerals such as magnesium and fulvic minerals to the filtered water before drinking it). I also suggest you find toothpastes and mouth rinses that do not have fluoride in them (at the end of the book I list some online sites where these things can be purchased). Avoid commercial baking powder, which may contain aluminum, as well, because when you mix the fluoride ion with aluminum it creates AlF3 (aluminum fluoride) which can readily penetrate your blood-brain barrier. Aluminum in the brain is not a good thing.

I have also installed fluoride-reducing showerhead filters, and I encourage you to do this as well. Even a shower filter that just filters out most of the chlorine in tap water is useful. When inorganic chlorine becomes vaporized, as it does during a shower, the chloroform in the vapor can be breathed in and chloroform may significantly increase your risk of developing cancer. Your skin is your largest organ, and according to the Extension Toxicology Network (EXTOXNET), "chemicals can be absorbed through skin and into the blood stream, causing toxic effects." The chlorine, bromine, and fluoride in municipal water can deplete your body of iodine, which can lead to hypothyroidism. According to Dr. Al Sears, almost 2 billion people are deficient in iodine. When I worked publically as a nutritional advisor, I saw many, many people (especially women) in their late 30s or early 40s who had "low energy" due to thyroid problems.

After significantly reducing the amount of fluoride and chlorine I was exposed to, I then researched how to reverse the calcification of my pineal gland (and my arteries) and found out EDTA (Ethylenediaminetetraacetic acid) worked for this. EDTA works by chelating (binding to and capturing) heavy metals and minerals and moving them out of your body via feces or urine. The first night I learned about EDTA I searched online until I found a place that sold this substance and was just about to buy some, but decided to wait. The VERY next night I hear on the radio that the Food and Drug Administration (FDA) was considering banning EDTA. I rushed to my computer and bought two large bottles [as of this writing, the FDA still have not banned it yet]. I did the EDTA chelation protocol three times (which simply involves taking 1 gram of EDTA for five days) and it worked! I could FEEL the difference!

EDTA will chelate many minerals out of your body. It will bind to and chelate toxic minerals like aluminum, fluoride, cadmium, lead, and mercury. It will also remove good stuff like copper, magnesium, and zinc. I would suggest you supplement with a good multi-mineral supplement immediately after finishing the chelation protocol. Ethylenediaminetetraacetic acid will remove calcium from atherosclerotic plaque but it does not cause calcium depletion (EDTA actually normalizes serum calcium levels by stimulating osteoblasts - the cells that make bone). EDTA has been shown to slow down the aging process. In one study, EDTA chelation therapy was found to increase the life span of female rats by almost 50% (Komarov, L.V., et al., 1983). It helps to reverse cross-linking (damage from free radicals) and in addition to improving the cardiovascular system (by helping to prevent calcium and cholesterol from forming into atherosclerotic plaque), it also helps the aforementioned pineal gland. EDTA may also help remove calcium deposits that make your blood vessels stiff and brittle, increase the blood flow to your heart and brain (giving them more oxygen and nutrients), and even fight wrinkles!

There are other credible, natural methods to decalcify your body that are worth mentioning but since I haven't tried them myself, I will just list them here:

Ingesting many lemons (high doses of citric acid have been shown to reduce calcium deposits)

Eating half a bulb of garlic every day for ten days (raw or cooked garlic contains active organosulfur compounds that may help prevent the kind of cholesterol that promotes calcium deposits)

Gazing at the sun for 15 minutes at sunrise and sunset (sunlight stimulates your pineal gland, but we'll talk more about that later)

Taking supplemental lysine and glutamic acid (because they may help you excrete calcium)

Visualizing a decalcified body and slowly saying "toe" in note C several times a day

A study done in 1997 demonstrated a natural way to reduce kidney stones. This study is relevant because kidneys stones are primarily calcium oxalate. In this study, Dr. Eric Braverman recommended using 1,000 milligrams (mg) of N-Acetyl-Cysteine (NAC), 1,000 mg of magnesium, 100 mg of vitamin B6, and 75 mg of potassium citrate each day for the prevention and treatment of kidney stones. Back when I worked as a public nutritionist, I remember hearing many kidney stone sufferers had been helped by this anti-calcium recipe. Chanca piedra, an herb native to South America, also helps to prevent kidney stones by inhibiting calcium oxalate crystals (Barros, M. E., et al, 2003).

Methods of GENERAL body detoxification include sweating toxins out through the use of infrared saunas or exercise, large doses of L-ascorbate (the best form of vitamin C), colon hydrotherapy, fasting, R-lipoic acid, magnesium citrate, chlorella, bentonite clay, fulvic minerals, astaxanthin, deep breathing exercises, and a diet consisting primarily of organic fruits and vegetables. Toxins and impurities in your body can actually reduce your life energy. After detoxifying your body properly, you should be able to hold more life force (chi, prana, ki ...etc.) in your body. Remember that analogy I mentioned about how you are like a radio receiver that needs to be powered up to receive a signal? Improving the health of your body is the first step to really powering yourself up to receive the signals that most people aren't even aware are being transmitted. I consider physical and mental detoxification and energizing your body to be prerequisites to being able to communicate with the Universe on a daily basis.

One final study regarding the pineal gland that I want to mention demonstrated food restriction slows the aging of the pineal gland and increases life span (Stokkan, K., et al., 1991). Rats that were kept on a food restriction diet (a very low calorie diet) had nearly twice the pineal and serum levels of both N-acetyltransferase (an endogenous enzyme manufactured within the pineal gland) and melatonin than rats that were allowed constant access to food had. This study also concluded aging in the rat is associated with a decrease in N-acetyltransferase and melatonin and the reason food restriction increases life span and reduces age-related physiological deterioration and diseases in many animals is due primarily to a healthier pineal gland.

Recommended supplements for pineal gland health include magnesium citrate, wheat germ, olive oil, pineapple juice, parsley, choline, and non-genetically engineered lecithin.

The [rife] frequency tone to activate your pineal gland is 936 Hz.

Chapter 8: The Amazing Benefits of Melatonin

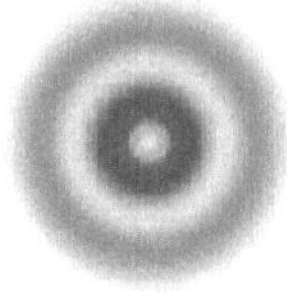

Most of the life-supporting properties of a healthy pineal gland are related to the gland's ability to produce melatonin (N-acetyl-5 methoxytryptamine). Melatonin is one of the very few molecules that is present in every plant and animal. While some melatonin is produced in your retina and gastrointestinal tract, your pineal gland is your main producer of this neurohormone (considered a neuropeptide). Melatonin has an incredible amount of health benefits. Part of the life-extending potential of this neurohormone is related to the idea it helps to maintain the health of mitochondria (the energy producers) in cells. Unlike other hormones, all the cells in your body have a receptor designed specifically to receive melatonin, which allows melatonin quick entry into all of your cells. Because of this, melatonin is considered an entire-body antioxidant. Several scientists have written in their clinical abstracts that melatonin seems to actually "communicate" directly with every one of your deoxyribonucleic acid (DNA) strands; many even suggest this "communication" includes "advice" on how the DNA can help the cell it resides in stay young and healthy. I wonder what other information could be communicated to every cell in your body via this mechanism?!

Melatonin may also:

Aid your cardiovascular system

Protect your brain from oxidation

Protect your cells and organs from damage (due to melatonin's antioxidant properties)

Help to reduce Irritable Bowel Syndrome (IBS) and indigestion symptoms

Help to heal ulcerative colitis and gastric ulcers

Help to prevent gallstones

Help protect your pancreas, liver, and kidneys from damage due to free radicals

Help to prevent macular degeneration (deteriorating eyesight), cataracts, and glaucoma

Help to increase HDL ("good") cholesterol levels

Help people suffering from chronic fatigue syndrome (CFS) correct their sleeping pattern

Almost double your number of activated immune cells (Maestroni, 1984)

Help to lower elevated blood sugar levels

Help obese people lose weight

Help your bones stay strong by supporting healthy osteoblasts (bone-cell makers)

Help your muscles relax

Help men reduce enlarged prostates and improve sexual performance

Help women experience less menopause symptoms

Help keep your skin healthy and alleviate and repair sunburns

Help counteract many, if not all, forms of cancer (at the dosage of 10-20 milligrams/day)

Reduce the impact of jet lag

...and don't forget it may very well help you live longer!

Melatonin helps your body become healthier and more energized and this kind of full-body energy isn't just something to help you get through your day. By increasing the health of your body, you are actually able to hold more of the life force in your body. In fact, it appears as though melatonin is able to increase the ability of every cell in your body to produce more energy.

I mentioned that I was "able to receive [divine] guidance on a daily basis," and I have had conversations with a being that "watches over me." The daily guidance I have been receiving occurs primarily at night when I have high levels of circulating melatonin and my brain is in a delta or theta brain wave state. I believe both the brain wave state and the melatonin play a role in my ability to receive these nightly downloads of information from the Universal Consciousness. I recommend you keep a pen and pad of paper near your bed (or get a digital recorder) and start keeping a journal of your dreams. Ask a question before you go to sleep and ask for assistance in finding the answer(s) to that question.

Raising the amount of energy in your body will help your body transmit signals further as well as receive them better. I believe melatonin helped me re-establish a dialogue with the off-world being that had originally contacted me in 1998. Shortly after purposefully raising my melatonin levels during daytime hours (which isn't normally advised), I was able to have a two-way conversation with this being again (after 13 years of not being able to speak with him while I was awake).

After several heartfelt requests on my part, this being agreed to tell me his name; it was a strange name with two hyphens in it. Later that day, when I typed this name into an internet search engine (without the hyphens) I learned there are some boys and men on this planet named this even though I had never heard of this name before. I was already certain this being was male as it emits energy I clearly read as "male" energy. I am strictly forbidden to tell others his name as he can "hear" it when people speak it with emotion and he doesn't have the ability to respond to millions of people calling out to him. He is NOT "God"; he informed me that he is not responsible for what happens in the majority of the Universe.

In my second conversation with this being, he told me I should "be very attentive to the things that I perceive to be under my care" and hinted that my level of caring for these things may determine the level of support I receive from the Universe. He also mentioned to me that humans should be especially careful how they treat other living things, especially other people and mammals. It was further suggested that beings of his nature disapprove of the way some people are treating beings that are so similar to ourselves [I no longer eat mammals]. He told me people should be caretakers of the earth and spoke about how the sun transmits energy to earth. He said he (and other beings) can send helpful instructions to everyone here, but **in order for a person to receive a significant amount of this information the person must desire to receive it, have faith in its existence, and be sensitive and aware enough to perceive the messages** (messages are being sent via different modalities, such as: words heard or seen, coincidences, intuitions, synchronicities, epiphanies achieved during times of high melatonin levels, during showers or other times you are well grounded, in dreams, and during meditation).

After imparting that knowledge on me, he then proceeded to encourage me to take better care of myself to serve others better. Shortly after this conversation, I learned to love myself consistently for the first time in at least 33 years. Not a selfish kind of love, but rather a deeply caring, forgiving state of allowance that permits the deep caring and "forgiving" of others as well. I came to realize that loving myself was to love all because all is one. I began the process of eradicating the belief I was apart or separate from other things. I was encouraged to become a "healthy, vibrantly alive [part of the Universe]" and to "give myself permission" to be joyful and pursue my dreams. I was told **beings of his nature want us to be healthy and happy**, but we have to both desire these things and consistently do what we intuitively know we should do to actualize that kind of reality for ourselves. Much of the information I receive from Source guides me towards increased health and an increased understanding of abilities that we already possess, and I am happy when I feel as though I am learning about these things and "moving forward."

In closing, he said, although he cares deeply for us and watches over this part of the Universe, he had several other obligations and told me in a nice way not to contact him (call out to him) unless it was a matter of momentous personal importance. Since I have most of my questions answered by nightly "downloads" of information, I have only contacted him once since this time. When I was in my twenties and thirties, I was quite restless and used to try to figure out the answers to all of life's seemingly impossible questions using "rational thought." I wasted a lot of time reading things, writing things down on paper, and trying to use my mind to figure out the nature of existence and what I should focus my time and energy on (if our minds could figure everything out we would all have nearly everything figured out by now). Nowadays, I feel very peaceful about virtually everything because every question I had about existence that I felt really needed to be answered has been answered.

In light of what this "watchoverer" told me, I believe when you ask the Universe for any kind of help you are, among other things, sending messages that a being (or beings) can actually receive. You may have to ask "the Universe" more than once, but what most people call "prayer" is real and absolutely works. Always exercise great humility and respect when speaking to beings that may be watching over you and feel and express gratitude for anything you ask for even before you are aware it has actualized in your reality. I would recommend routinely sending out love and thanks to those who might be watching over you.

It is important to remember, however, that YOU are a powerful creator, and you are the one who creates your own reality. Let what is already a part of your HIGHER SELF emerge by listening to your heart and truly BEING YOU in every way. In future books in this series I will talk much more about how to prevent yourself from consciously or unconsciously suppressing the true YOU to conform to societal pressures or submit to other people's limiting beliefs.

Personally, I don't fear malicious spirits or beings because I can sense energy and I feel as though I have protection from negative energies, but you should always exercise caution when asking for assistance from external beings. Ask them directly if they are from the light and are here to help you because even mischievous beings are sometimes unable to lie about these things. Reiterate that you are asking for the best possible guide available that will help you achieve higher good for both yourself and others. Although feelings of overwhelm and personal inadequacy are to be expected when first being contacted, if you don't feel compassion from the being, command it to go away and do not allow it to become a part of your life.

Chapter 9: How to Enhance Melatonin Levels

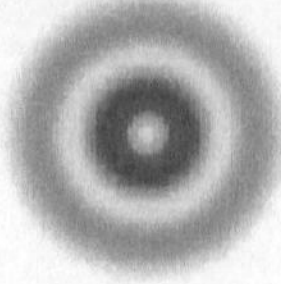

Virtually all the things that are good for your pineal gland are good for proper melatonin production. There are, however, several specific ways to increase the amount of melatonin in your body.

The first thing to realize about your melatonin level is that it's subject to dramatic natural fluctuations throughout the circadian (24-hour day) rhythm. You produce melatonin during the daytime but your melatonin level is low because you don't secrete it (light prevents the daytime secretion of norepinephrine). When you're in darkness, the melatonin level in your bloodstream usually begins to increase because your pineal gland starts secreting the melatonin it has produced during the daylight hours.

The nighttime peak in your melatonin level usually shortens as the days grow longer, so people tend to have longer periods of peak melatonin in the winter. Melatonin usually reaches its peak at around 2 AM in young people and around 3 AM in older people. Another fact to be aware of is that people under 18 years of age usually have plenty of melatonin and people over 45 usually have very little.

Sunlight stimulates your pineal gland to produce melatonin, where it is stored for nighttime release. Although the production of melatonin is actually regulated by the pattern of your suprachiasmatic nucleus (SCN), not the darkness itself, too much nighttime light on your eyes causes your suprachiasmatic nucleus to inhibit the release of melatonin.

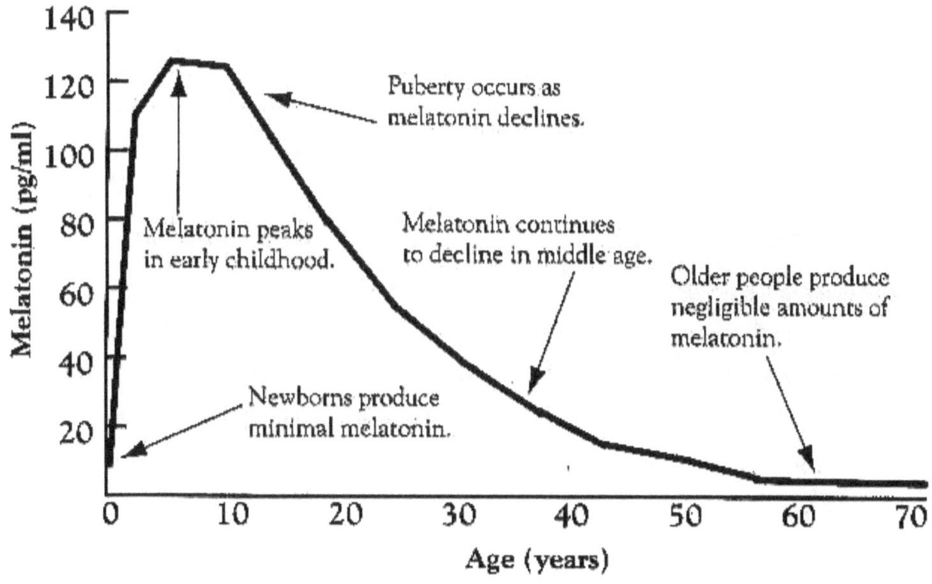

Melatonin listed in picograms per milliliter of blood.
A picogram is a trillionth of a gram.
Figure credit: *Melatonin* by Dr. Russel J. Reiter

Because sunlight (and similar light spectrums) can stimulate melatonin production, one important method of increasing melatonin production is to allow more light to enter the retinas of your eyes. Studies have already demonstrated that as little as half an hour of light therapy (heliotherapy or photobiology) a day can "cure" about 75% of people suffering from Seasonal Affective Disorder (SAD) (Gallin, P. F., et al., 1995). Most researchers believe it is sunlight's ability to stimulate melatonin production in the pineal gland that accounts for this improvement in those suffering from seasonal depression. The invisible, ultraviolet bands of light excite epithelial cells in the retina, which transmit the stimulus through the optic nerve to the pituitary and pineal glands.

According to Daniel Reid's wonderful book *The Tao of Health, Sex & Longevity*, "Taoists adepts realized the medical benefits of sunlight thousands of years ago. *The Tao Tsang* (*Treasury of Tao*), compiled over 2,000 years ago, contains numerous references to heliotherapy, which it refers to as 'the method of administering sunbeams'. It advises exposing both the naked body and the naked eyes directly to sunlight to assimilate vital solar energy. It states unequivocally that exposing the eyes to direct sunlight greatly 'benefits the brain' by stimulating secretions of 'vital essence' there." He goes on to state that although Western medicine has just recently recognized the method through which sunlight stimulates melatonin production (and labeled it the "oculo-endocrine system"), this "mechanism has been known to Taoists for ages." Mr. Reid also states when "full-spectrum light" is restored to your retinas, your pituitary gland, which is the "master regulator of the endocrine system," secretes its vital hormones into your bloodstream. Be aware that glass, glasses, or contact lenses significantly reduce the amount of ultraviolet rays reaching your retinas.

Many people wear sunglasses and apply sunscreen because they believe the sun is harmful to their eyes and skin. While it's true that overexposure to the sun can cause damage to your skin and is a factor in developing cataracts, I suspect many, many more people are causing harm to themselves by not getting enough sunlight. Besides the fact most "suntan lotions" contain a toxic cocktail of chemical ingredients that can be absorbed through your skin, it is my personal belief that getting about 20 minutes of direct sunlight between the hours of 10 am and noon is a powerful and important way for me to energize my entire physical body. I also believe some sunlight on my eyes is good for them (for one thing I've seen studies that strongly suggest melatonin helps to prevent cataracts and glaucoma and sunlight on your retinas helps to produce melatonin). I never stare directly at the sun, but I do the Tibetan eye exercises around the sun (see http://www.wakingtimes.com/2013/04/19/tibetan-exercises-for-eye-health/ for more details). If I had not purposefully moved to a warm, sunny place on this earth I would have probably purchased an indoor "sunlamp" by now. Sun exposure is critical to maintaining a healthy endogenous vitamin D level, and Dr. Joseph Mercola estimates that approximately 70% of Americans have low vitamin D levels. According to Dr. Mercola, "Regularly spending even relatively short intervals of only 10 to 15 minutes in the sunlight allows your body to produce vitamin D, and having adequate vitamin D3 levels can drastically reduce your risk of colon and breast cancer." He continues, stating that researchers "from the Moore's Cancer Center at the University of California, San Diego (UCSD), estimated that by increasing vitamin D3 levels, particularly in countries north of the equator, 250,000 cases of colorectal cancer, and 350,000 cases of breast cancer could be prevented worldwide. In all, that amounts to 600,000 cases of breast and colorectal cancer prevented, including close to 150,000 in the U.S. alone." Vitamin D may also ward off many other illnesses due to the fact it can strengthen your immune system. A recent study reported that people deficient in vitamin D had a 164% higher morbidity rate (Vacek, J, 2012). For more details on the benefits of sun exposure visit: http://www.mercola.com/Downloads/bonus/benefits-of-sun-exposure/report.htm.

In the first few months of 2012, there were a few days when I felt as though I was being bombarded with information from "above." I was getting so much information, even during my waking hours, that I felt as light-headed as if I were drinking alcohol. Fortunately, I soon realized I was only feeling this way approximately two days after the sun had produced a coronal mass ejection (what many people call a "solar flare"). The magnetic fields in the sun can twist and snap, producing explosions of plasma and charged particles that have a force millions of times what they claim hydrogen bombs can produce. Plasma is the fourth state of matter (solid, liquid, gas, plasma). While light emitted from the sun only takes about 8 minutes to reach the earth, it takes about 30 to 72 hours for plasma and charged particles released from the sun to reach the earth. Plasma is an ionized gas that is so powerful that it is able to free electrons from atoms or molecules. Plasma may be the most common state of matter in the universe. I believe I was receiving some information from these charged particles the sun was emitting. What if all sunlight contains information? Imagine if the sun was constantly emitting information. What if sunlight is able to deliver information to your optic nerve that is then transmitted to your pineal gland and other parts of your brain? What if your pineal gland is able to imprint this information into the melatonin it produces and that melatonin communicates that information directly to every cell of your body when it communicates with the DNA in every cell of your body?

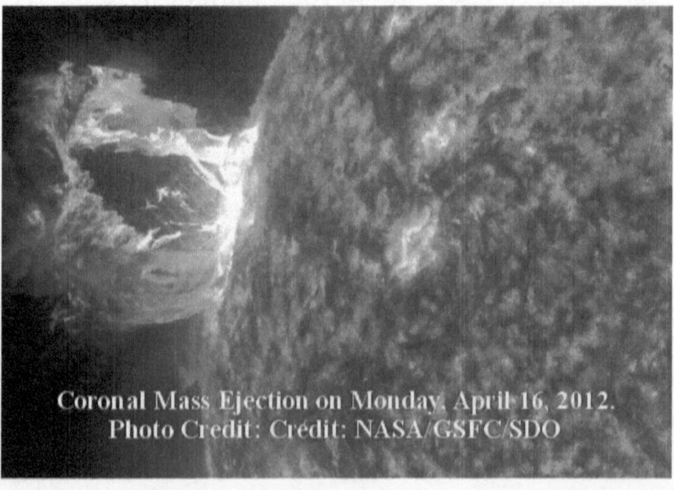

Coronal Mass Ejection on Monday, April 16, 2012.
Photo Credit: Credit: NASA/GSFC/SDO

Some people fear these "solar storms" and the resulting EMF (electric and magnetic fields) they produce. In addition to the very real possibility that a powerful EMF pulse could knock the electrical grid offline (which would cause almost all financial transactions to stop and water pumps to stop functioning), EMF's may alter melatonin production and heart function (Masami Ishido, et al., 2001, Dubbels, R. 1986, Stoupel, et al., 1996). The sun affects the electromagnetic field of the earth and the earth's electromagnetic field affects our personal (auric) electromagnetic field. Man-made EMF's, such as those generated by electric motors, electric blankets, "smart" meters, wireless phones, cell phones, cell towers, and routers can also interfere with our personal energetic fields. I put my wireless router on a timer that turns it off at night, and I don't sleep next to any electrical devices (I've noticed that when the router is left on my dreams tend to revolve around physical density subjects and when I have it off I am much more apt to dream creatively and receive answers). I don't want any human-made signal interfering with my receiving of any non-man-made signals.

Let me give you an example of a time I picked up some information "out of thin air." The information itself is about as trivial as you can imagine, but this particular event proved to me that the "psychic" abilities I seemed to be developing were real. One morning I woke up and there was one thing on my mind: margarine. I don't eat margarine, nor does anyone in my house, and I couldn't even tell you the last time I had seen or heard the word or product margarine; it was probably quite a long time since I usually don't even shop at stores that sell margarine and this was before I started writing my nutrition book that describes in detail how unhealthy hydrogenated fat is. Anyway, I was thinking about how unhealthy margarine is, how it's chemically quite similar to plastic, how it's high in trans fats (hydrogenated oil - ick!), and how it increases the risk of cancer (all of which I knew because I worked as a nutritionist). Then I thought about the fact I ate it as a child because my father was told by his doctor that it was good for him and his high cholesterol. Then I thought, "Hmm, I wonder if my dad knows now how unhealthy margarine is … I'm not sure I ever told him about this." Soon thereafter, I go downstairs and power up my laptop to view my emails. There's a new email right on top entitled "Pass the butter please." I open the email and quickly realize the email is a "chain letter" type email which is describing how unhealthy margarine is, specifically how it is [according to the email] "one molecule away from being plastic," is "very high in trans fatty acids," and "increases the risk of cancers up to five times." The email is from my dad who had sent it to me while I was sleeping that morning (he's on east coast time, I'm on west coast time). I only receive about one email a month from my dad and it's usually about some specific, poignant matter, and virtually never a chain letter. Hmm…

Besides getting daily, full-spectrum light, it has been established that food restriction can significantly preserve melatonin levels in aging mammals. Other strategies to raise your pineal gland's production of melatonin levels include relaxation, visualization, meditation, and the use of focused electromagnetic energy. Dark blue fruits, spices, and mantras have been used to help stimulate the power and production of your "third eye chakra" area. Air, incense, and herbs can stimulate your "crown chakra" and chi gung can get all of your chakras energized. My friend, Vicki Howie, makes temporary tattoos called "Chakra Booster Healing Tattoos" that help bring energy to your chakras.

It has also been demonstrated that exogenous (not made in the body but rather supplemental) melatonin can help one's body in similar ways to endogenous (produced in the body) melatonin.

Generally, however, it is not advisable for people under the age of 30 to take melatonin supplements every day because studies have shown that young mice receiving daily doses of exogenous melatonin have shortened life spans. Children and teenagers should not supplement with melatonin nor should anyone with severe allergies. Other people who should be wary of taking melatonin supplements are those taking supplemental cortisone, monoamine oxidase (MAO) inhibitors, and selective serotonin reuptake inhibitors (SSRI's). In addition, exogenous melatonin should not be used by pregnant or lactating women because studies have not yet proven this is safe.

If you choose to take melatonin supplements on a regular basis, you should take them at the same time each day, usually directly before the time you usually sleep. The recommended dosages can vary widely between individuals; some people, including me, achieve good results with as little as 0.1 milligram (mg), but most melatonin users take between 1 mg and 10 mg per night. Melatonin is considered extremely safe and non-toxic, but you may experience drowsiness the next day if you take a dose that is too high for you. Be aware melatonin is extremely powerful, and you probably have less than 10 picograms of melatonin circulating in your blood (1,000,000,000 picograms = 1 milligram). For anti-aging purposes, a daily dosage range of 0.1 mg (low end) to 3.0 mg (upper end) is recommended (Reiter, R. 1996). Supplemental melatonin has not been shown to reduce your body's natural production of melatonin and most people sleep better when taking supplemental melatonin. Melatonin supplements, even ones produced in laboratories, are chemically identical to endogenously produced melatonin. I would choose a time-released (sustained release) melatonin product over one that releases the dosage all at once.

As a nutritionist, I have always believed a healthy body knows what hormones to produce, when to produce them and how much of them to produce. Consequently, I have never been a strong advocate of taking supplemental hormones. For example, people taking large dosages of human growth hormone (hGH) can damage their pancreas. If they worked together with their bodies, they could raise their hGH naturally by carefully making the vitamins, amino acids, and other precursors of hGH available to their pituitary gland. Now in the case of melatonin we have a substance that is considered more of an antioxidant than a hormone by perhaps its premier researcher, Dr. Russel Reiter. I take supplemental antioxidants every day. Furthermore, we have evidence that our primary melatonin makers, our pineal glands, may have been damaged by environmental factors that we have been subjected to. The bottom line is, since I believe melatonin is very good for my body, facilitates my enlightenment, and is declining as I get older; I have been exploring ways to assist my body's natural ability to manufacture melatonin.

Several foods contain melatonin. Rice (both white and brown) and oats have about 1 to 1.8 nanograms of melatonin per gram (1,000,000 nanograms = 1 milligram). Montmorency cherries contain approximately 13.46 nanograms of melatonin per gram (Burkhardt S, Reiter RJ, et al., 2001).

In addition to eating certain foods, there are natural supplements you can take to encourage endogenous melatonin production. One of my favorite approaches when deciding which supplements to take to support a certain function in my body is to put supplements I already know are good for me at the top of the list. B vitamins are water-soluble and your body is unable to store them, so I know I need to ingest them daily. Folic acid (a B vitamin) is required for your body to make melatonin. Vitamins B3, B6, and B12 also help your body manufacture melatonin. Although it's always best to obtain nutrition via your diet, a good whole-food multi-vitamin or "B-Complex 100" supplement can technically provide all these vitamins. In addition to boosting your immune system, zinc can raise melatonin levels. Taking magnesium citrate and a small amount of calcium citrate right before you go to sleep can help you produce melatonin. The vast majority of people are deficient in magnesium (approximately 85%) and your body uses magnesium to relax your muscles. When your muscles are relaxed, your mind actually becomes less tense, which is why I recommend anyone suffering from stress take supplemental magnesium citrate (see *The Complete Anxiety and Panic Attack Cure*" book for more details). My research has come up with a simple formula for figuring out how much supplemental magnesium to take: Take 2 milligrams of magnesium citrate for every pound you weigh, each day, and never take more calcium than magnesium (odds are your calcium to magnesium ratio in your body is too high). I get periodic blood tests to check the vitamin and mineral levels in my body and I encourage you to do the same.

Another thing you need to put into your body daily is protein, because, like B vitamins, it cannot be stored in your body. Protein is composed of amino acids and all protein sources such as meat, eggs, and dairy products contain amino acids. Perhaps the most important amino acid in relation to melatonin production is tryptophan. Your body converts tryptophan into 5-hydroxytryptophan (5-HTP), and your body can convert 5-HTP into serotonin, n-acetyl serotonin, and eventually into melatonin. Therefore, taking 5-hydroxytryptophan and/or tryptophan may increase your melatonin levels. The supplement known as SAMe (S-Adenosylmethionine) can help turn your serotonin into melatonin. Finally, methionine (an amino acid) and acetyl-l-carnitine (ALC) may help both your gastrointestinal tract (where some melatonin is produced) and your pineal gland produce melatonin.

In addition to these body-friendly vitamins and minerals, some herbs have been shown to increase the amount of melatonin produced in your pineal gland. Saint John's Wort can dramatically increase the amount of serotonin in your body and serotonin can be turned into melatonin. There is one herb, however, that will boost your melatonin levels higher than any other substance known to humankind (other than straight melatonin): cannabis. In a study performed in 1986, it was shown that cannabis (also known as marijuana or "pot") may be able to raise melatonin levels by approximately 4,000% (Lissoni, P., Resentini, M., and Fraschini, F.). The right amount of cannabis at the right time could be beneficial for your body. Back when I worked as a public nutritionist, people would often ask me if smoking cannabis was harmful to their health. After researching the topic, I discovered there were studies that showed that smoking cannabis might not be harmful to your body. A study done by Donald Tashkin in 2006 showed that, although the smoke from burned cannabis has some potentially cancer-causing substances in it, one of the ingredients in cannabis smoke, delta-9-tetrahydrocannabinol (Δ-9-THC usually referred to as THC) may protect your body from cancer by killing cancer cells. Tashkin's study, funded by the National Institute on Drug Abuse, studied over 2,000 people and found no increased incidence of cancer in people who smoked cannabis regularly.

A more recent study, conducted by Mark Pletcher of the University of California, examined the effects smoking cigarettes and marijuana had on over 5,000 people over the course of twenty years. These results, which were published in the January 11, 2012 edition of Journal of the American Medical Association, concluded that smoking one cannabis cigarette (a joint) every day for seven years was associated with a slight

INCREASE in lung airflow rates and an INCREASE in lung capacity. The study also concluded the more tobacco one smokes the more lung capacity and airflow DECREASED. Unlike commercial tobacco, the vast majority of cannabis does not contain added chemicals to help it stay lit or taste differently.

Some cannabis users use a heating device called a "vaporizer" to heat the herb to a temperature that is high enough to liberate the desirable compounds present in the plant matter without releasing potentially toxic elements. For example, the boiling point of delta-9-tetrahydrocannabinol (Δ-9-THC) is approximately 314.6 °F (157 °C), the boiling point of cannabidiol (CBD) is approximately 356 °F (180 °C), the boiling point of delta-8-tetrahydrocannabinol (Δ-8-THC) is approximately 352 °F (178 °C), and the boiling point of cannabinol (CBN) is approximately 365 °F (185 °C). This means one could heat the herb to approximately 370 °F and receive all those elements without taking in significant amounts of potential carcinogens such as benzene, which has a boiling point of approximately 392 °F (200 °C). When you light the cannabis herb on fire, you are exposing the plant material to temperatures around 1100 °F (593 °C) which may indeed release several carcinogens. The only toxin present In the vapor of cannabis subjected to a temperature of 370 °F, that I am aware of, is toluene. Toluene can irritate the nose and throat and cause dizziness and headaches. Interestingly enough, melatonin helps to counteract toluene toxicity due to its antioxidative properties (Pascual, R., et al., 2010), and cannabis helps to stimulate melatonin production. Some cannabis users make "cannabutter" by simmering the herb in melted butter for several hours and then they eat the butter along with some food or as part of a recipe. It's hard even for me to think of cannabis as a vegetable after all the lies and misinformation I've heard about the herb over the years, but cannabis is a plant.

Furthermore, I have never seen a single reputable study that showed even moderately heavy cannabis usage causes any significant brain damage. In fact, Dr. Igor Grant, the Executive Vice Chairman at the University of California, San Diego Department of Psychiatry, who conducted one of the largest studies exploring the effects of heavy marijuana use on people's brains, wrote:

"Smoking marijuana will certainly affect perception, but it does not cause permanent brain damage. The findings were kind of a surprise. One might have expected to see more impairment of higher mental function. Other illegal drugs, or even alcohol, can cause brain damage."

Most scientists believe the primary "brain stimulating" ingredient in smoked cannabis is the aforementioned delta-9-tetrahydrocannabinol. THC merely temporarily binds to and activates specific receptors in the brain known as cannabinoid receptors. These receptors are there because your body produces its own endocannabinoids such as anandamide and 2-arachidonoylglycerol.

Getting "high" on cannabis is not without any risk, however. Cannabis can inhibit your normal thought patterns, which can affect short-term memory and your ability to think in a linear fashion. One should never alter their consciousness before driving a car or operating heavy machinery. Cannabis can temporarily change how your mind focuses, impair motor skills, and can cause you to react more slowly to unexpected events. Still, after I have examined many studies that have been conducted on the effects of cannabis on the health of people, I have no compelling evidence to induce me to tell my clients that marijuana is definitely hazardous to their health. In fact, I began to wonder why the herb has been made illegal in most parts of the world. I have never seen or heard of a single confirmed case where cannabis killed anyone, yet we all know that alcohol and tobacco, which are legal, essentially kill many people.

Chapter 10: The Effects of Cannabis and Dimethyltryptamine (DMT) on Enlightenment

Marijuana has been used by many famous artists and creators over the years. Many of these people claim that smoking cannabis has increased their creativity, allowed them to compose music easier, or inspired them to invent something fantastic. One remarkable person who admitted smoking cannabis on a regular basis is the late Carl Sagan. Mr. Sagan was an astronomer, astrophysicist, cosmologist, scientist, and author of over 600 literary documents. An excerpt from an essay that he composed under the pseudonym "Mr. X" reads as follows:

"I do not consider myself a religious person in the usual sense, but there is a religious aspect to some [cannabis] highs. The heightened sensitivity in all areas gives me a feeling of communion with my surroundings, both animate and inanimate. Sometimes a kind of existential perception of the absurd comes over me and I see with awful certainty the hypocrisies and posturing of myself and my fellow men. And at other times, there is a different sense of the absurd, a playful and whimsical awareness. Both of these senses of the absurd can be communicated, and some of the most rewarding highs I've had have been in sharing talk and perceptions and humor. Cannabis brings us an awareness that we spend a lifetime being trained to overlook and forget and put out of our minds." Later in the essay he says he is "convinced that there are genuine and valid levels of perception available with cannabis (and probably with other drugs) which are, through the defects of our society and our educational system, unavailable to us without such drugs."

Mr. Sagan wrote that smoking cannabis "has produced a very rich array of insights," and "the devastating insights achieved when high are real insights." He expressed a serious sentiment in a hyperbolic manner when he wrote "ten even more interesting ideas or images have to be lost in the effort of recording one. It is easy to understand why someone might think it's a waste of effort going to all that trouble to set the thought down."

I know what he's talking about. Imagine waking up in the morning and immediately realizing that some amazing, new thoughts are in the forefront of your mind, thoughts you had never consciously thought before. These thoughts are so unique, insightful, and paradigm shifting that you feel compelled to rush over to grab a pen and piece of paper so you can write these ideas down. Imagine if these thoughts didn't originate in your mind but rather were some kind of "information download" you received directly from a higher mind or consciousness. Well, this event happens to me nearly every morning! After writing the ideas down, I pause to reflect on them and the personal meaning they have for me. Usually the ideas are essentially telling me to change an aspect of my reality and I usually rush out of my bedroom eager to actualize a better reality for myself and others. These divine ideas come complete with the energy to make them a reality, and I know they're the right ideas for me because I feel they were gifted directly to me. The Universe doesn't make mistakes! The things the Universe recommends to you are ideas you can conceive and achieve ... in fact it's RELYING ON YOU to actualize those ideas in this physical dimension (bring more of YOU into this reality).

I believe your expectations are important. If you smoke marijuana just to get high, you will get high; if you smoke marijuana to receive guidance and epiphanies you will receive guidance and epiphanies. If you believe life is a struggle, it will be a struggle; if you think life is wonderful it, will be wonderful. For example, you can be happy almost all the time by deciding to be happy all the time. Happiness is a state of mind that you control. Happiness doesn't have to be contingent on any external factors; happiness is a choice.

It occurred to me that the state I'm in when receiving nightly transmissions from the Universe and the state Mr. Sagan was describing have a huge thing in common: They're both states characterized by high melatonin levels.

Some people believe the reason cannabis is illegal is because it poses a threat to the very powerful companies that control the oil, cotton, soybean, corn, alcohol, tobacco, and pharmaceutical industries. Hemp, which is a variety of cannabis, can be made into food, fuel, paper, textiles, and clothing. Other people believe the reason cannabis is illegal is because it creates huge money allotments for law enforcement agencies, lawyers, prisons, and courts. Some people are convinced the reason cannabis is illegal is because it may cause enlightenment and the powers that be don't want a population that is very awake and aware (the same reason why they put fluoride in the water?). Maybe the reason cannabis is illegal in most places is a mixture of all of these factors, but as far as I'm concerned the reason cannabis is illegal is NOT because it's harmful to your body or causes you to segue into harder drugs (the "gateway drug" theory).

Before I started researching the facts about our pineal glands, I fully expected to write quite a bit about a tryptamine alkaloid known as dimethyltryptamine (DMT) in this book. I had heard

DMT was produced by your pineal gland and was a powerful psychedelic drug capable of bridging the gap between everyday physical reality and the spirit realm. Well, here's the problem: it has never been proven that dimethyltryptamine is produced in the pineal gland or anywhere else in the brain. In all likelihood, a small amount of DMT probably is produced in your brain, but you're not going to be able to stimulate your body to produce enough endogenous dimethyltryptamine to give you enlightenment.

Nonetheless, dimethyltryptamine is a naturally occurring substance found in various plants and animals and in small quantities in the human brain. DMT has been extracted from plants and used as a drug for over 4,000 years. The indigenous people in South America often consume DMT during shamanic rituals. This is done by combining DMT-containing plant material with a monoamine oxide inhibitor and the resulting product is called ayahuasca (pronounced ah-yuh-wah-skuh). Ayahuasca refers to any of the various psychoactive preparations derived from the banisteriopsis caapi vine mixed with the leaves of dimethyltryptamine-containing plant species from the genus psychotria.

The strong effects of concentrated DMT ingestion (or inhalation) include the feelings of being transported to a completely different place, being immersed in kaleidoscopic sounds and images, and/or being in communication with spirit entities. Some people believe DMT is capable of tuning the brain to the frequencies of other dimensions, like tuning a radio to a particular radio station. I believe I must raise the vibration of my personal energy field to communicate with certain entities (the entities actually slow their vibrations down to facilitate the exchange of information). It's interesting to think there may be other dimensions all around us that we are simply out of vibrational synchronization with and do not detect with our three-dimensional senses. In addition, once you have actually experienced the feeling of transcending this reality it is easier for you to do so again.

Many users of dimethyltryptamine report that the beings they met and/or the experiences they had with the help of the drug caused their entire perspective on life to change. Like cannabis, DMT can strip away lies that we tell ourselves and remove limitations that our minds are conditioned to defend. DMT can force you to face your reality in a starker manner. This insight may reveal aspects of your personality or character that are not in line with your true, higher self, which can help you to choose to act and be truer to the "real" you in the future.

What I find especially interesting about this drug is some users claim they are actually able to receive detailed instructions on how to heal people (usually using plants) by spirit beings. For more information on dimethyltryptamine please reference the book (or movie) called *DMT: The Spirit Molecule* by Dr. Rick Strassman.

Chapter 11: Increasing the Amount of Joy in Your Life

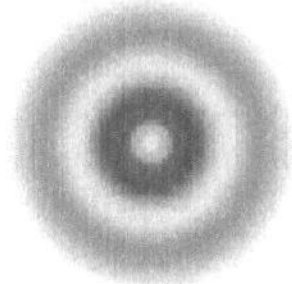

Here's a list of things that can help give you more joy and the more joy you have the easier they will be to do:

Abandon anger

Reduce the level of stress in your life

Be resilient and flexible

Work well with others

Become more grateful

Keep your heart healthy

Reduce conflict

Choose a fantastic mood

Erase fears

Relax your body and muscles

Abandon defensiveness

Recharge your energy

Strengthen relationships

Count your blessings

Smile

Boost your immunity

Develop your spirituality

Decrease pain

Add zest to life

Reduce anxiety

Release inhibitions

Be spontaneous

See things in a humorous light

Attract others to yourself

Laugh

Stay present and live for today. Don't let the past or future cloud your mind. All you have to do today is make it to your bed tonight. Ask yourself, "Do I really need __________ for me to be content right now?"

The trick is to remember that you wish to remain in a state of joy and not return to the default states of worry, fear, or numbness that many people seem to spend much of their time in. Amazingly enough, even though people have the ability to gift themselves happiness, they often choose not to. Instead of engaging in activities that they find genuinely joyful they watch the nightly news, or worry about money, or hurt their body by believing that they have cancer. I don't watch the news because the mainstream media doesn't usually report on the things that are important to me, and when they do, they sometimes say things that are something other than The Truth. I don't worry much about money because I'm a minimalist who's grateful for what I have, which allows me to live in a state of abundance. When you have gratitude and give thanks for something, you are instructing the Universe to give you more of that thing. The amount of money you allow yourself to command is related to how much personal power you allow yourself to establish. I don't view most diseases as anything that can stand up against nature's cures. Much of what is defined as "disease" is directly connected to the stagnation of body energies. People can shorten their lifespans considerably just by believing the doctor who tells them they have a terminal condition or by focusing on average lifespan data. Most people marinate in the lower energies of anger, fear, worry, desire, and sorrow or engage in unhelpful thoughts of pride, superiority, or fantasy futures that they don't even believe are possible. Why do they continue to do that? They do it because those levels of being, those vibrational energies, are so familiar to them that they find those feelings comfortable and reassuring. They have defined themselves by those levels of body energy and the thoughts associated with those body energy vibrations. [Please don't let my use of the terms "energy" or "vibration" bother you; I am merely very aware of the fact that EVERYTHING is actually energy. If you don't believe me, ask a quantum scientist next time you meet one. Seriously, though, if you accept the idea that matter is made out of atoms then you should be aware that, at a quantum level, there appears to be almost nothing "physically" there inside atoms. As far as we can tell, an atom is over 99% immaterial but is full of energy.] Many people actually think that the person that they have been in the past **is** them and they couldn't possibly change themselves into something amazing in this lifetime. Most people have become so defensive of their beliefs, way of doing things, and labels that others have labeled them with, that they habitually return to their old way of being and their set routines even though they realize on some level that doing so is detrimental to their own health and happiness; anything outside of their current paradigm is routinely rejected. The ironic thing is that their salvation lies in the thoughts that they would immediately label as "illogical." Perhaps the most common regret people have at the end of their lives is that they never lived in a manner that honored their true, unique selves and they never found the courage to pursue their dreams. Sadly, many people are so afraid of change and the unknown consequences change might bring with it that they avoid moving out of their comfort coffins. The last thing they want to do is feel more responsible for their situation. In all likelihood, you have conditioned yourself to remain in some of these lower energies. Establish new pathways to happiness by smiling often and consistently remembering to choose happiness. Form some new "neural grooves" in your brain by consistently performing joyous actions and forming new neural pathways. Just as more freeways head toward the places with the most activity, it's believed that habitual thought patterns start physically "wiring" your brain to return to those habitual thought patterns. Having a fear arise periodically is natural but moving forward in spite of fear is bravery. Be brave and take action. Consistent positive action gives you faith in yourself. Faith dispels fear.

Thank you for being an aware person trying to improve yourself and much peace, joy, and love to you!

It may be difficult to find EDTA or fluoride-free products in your local area. You can find these items online at Vitacost.com or iherb.com.

You can find several videos I made discussing various topics related to health and spirituality on YouTube under my username BrightLightSite.

Please feel free to email me at jblanchard3000@yahoo.com. I would love to hear from you! Please contact me if you have any information for me, questions for me, would like to interview or quote me, or would like to receive an email to notify you when my next book is released.

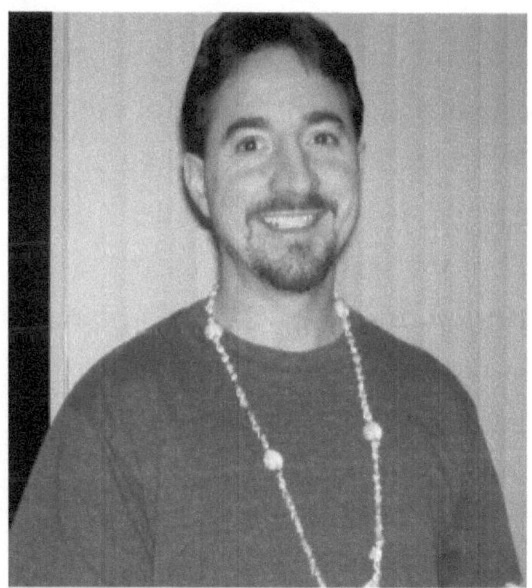

Special thanks to Dr. Russel J. Reiter for corresponding with me and allowing me to reference his vast knowledge.

Photo and Figure Credits

Pineal Gland diagram courtesy of http://www.fluoridealert.org

Descarte's woodcut photo courtesy of
www.princeton.eduDescartes

Fluoride toxicity chart courtesy of
http://www.lovethetruth.com/truth_about_floride.htm